Overcome Insomnia

19 Natural Ways To Overcome Insomnia

Joan Ali

Disclaimer

Care has been taken to ensure that the information in this eBook is accurate to the best of my knowledge. The reader should understand that the information provided in this eBook does not contain legal, medical or any kind of professional advice.

Just to let you know that I am neither a doctor nor do I consider myself to be one. I am not liable for mis- statements, omissions or inaccurate information. This book is for informational use and is not intended to treat, diagnose or cure any illness. Should you choose to use any of this information for yourself, your child or anyone else I recommend you do so by first consulting with your medical practitioner? This product has no warranties. Following the suggestions in this book is done at your own risk. The information provided in this eBook is not intended to substitute for medical advice from a health care professional.

Please consult your doctor if you have any symptoms stated in this eBook or suffer from any medical condition. This eBook should not be used for diagnosing or treating health problems.

The author and publisher shall have neither responsibility nor liability to any person or entity with respect to any damage caused or alleged to be caused directly or indirectly by this eBook.

Contents

Thanks for downloading this book.

To obtain a good night's sleep is every human being intention, yet so few of us really get a good night sleep for various reasons.

In this book you will learn the importance of sleep and how a lack of it can affect your health relationships and other aspects of your life. It covers the causes and symptoms of sleeplessness, the types of insomnia, stages of sleep, sleep study, medications and its side effects, supplements, simple changes that can help, acupressure, meditation, teas, sleep environment and many other natural therapies to help you achieve a good night sleep.

You will find that you already have some of these things in your kitchen or bathroom and with some simple changes that will not cost you anything you may start sleeping your best.

There are several different ways in this book that will help with your insomnia. You do not have to use them all; one person may only need to make a simple change that will help them to overcome insomnia whereas others may need to incorporate more than one therapy to accomplish the same benefit. What you will find is that there is something to help most people.

Many More than 70 million people in the United States suffer from chronic sleep disorders that can be treated according to The U.S. Institute of Health.

Americans are plagued by sleepless nights many of them either work very long hours, some to provide for their families others to climb the corporate ladder at a very steep price. Others to take care of babies or ailing family members. There are also those who love to watch TV, movies, play video games, emails and use electronic devices till the early hours of the morning.

After several sleepless nights your body becomes very tired and unable to function properly putting you at risk for accidents at the work place, at home or even while driving. People who drive without getting a good night sleep fall asleep while they are driving. They become very moody and hard to get along with during this time. They snap at their family members and others for no apparent reason. Yet when these people get a good night sleep they seem like a different person altogether.

Sleep is very important for your health so everyone should try their best to get a good night sleep.

There are so many people who sacrifice many sleepless nights and their families and survive on 3 to 4 hours of sleep because they want to climb the corporate ladder; by the time some of them get there, they have already lost their families because they had no time to spend with them. Others just want to go out and have fun till 3 or 4am then get up at 7 to go to work, yet others stay up till 1 or 2 in the morning playing computer games, watching TV or sending emails.

Still there are people who will pay someone any amount of money to get a good night's sleep. Sleep medications and supplements are big business. Americans spend about $2 billion dollars a year on prescription medicines. You do not have to pay a bill to go to sleep yet that is what millions of Americans are doing. This is FREE. Everyone is looking for a quick fix so they end up spending their money for it.

Estimated cost for loss productivity to U.S. employers is approximately $18 billion dollars a year.

What is Insomnia

General insomnia is when a person has trouble falling asleep, staying asleep, or waking up too early even if they have the time to sleep. These disorders may also be defined by an overall poor quality of sleep. Sleep is essential to everyone's health, wellbeing, mind and mood. Therefore everyone should try to get a good night sleep.

The benefits of sleep.

Insomnia is a very common complaint, but it is not a sleep disorder. Insomnia is most likely a symptom of a medical problem or being overload with responsibilities which varies with each individual.

Sleep is very important for our health so when we sleep the body can repair itself, tissues and muscles can be rebuilt and restored. Growth hormone is also secreted during this time. Growth hormone is very important for children who are growing and also in adults. It also restores the body's energy supply that was depleted during the day.

You should get at least seven or eight hours of sleep every night, although some people feel great after five hours of sleep. Even this is not always possible you should try.

Studies have shown that getting a good night sleep can prevent you from getting some serious health problems such as:

High blood pressure

Heart disease

Stroke

Heart attacks

Obesity

Better sex life

May help reduce pain

Lower your risk of accidents

Lower your risk of fall/injury

Puts you in a better mood

Stronger immunity

You will be able to make better decisions

Help you to solve problems better

Healthy weight

Lower stress

Avoid accidents

Help prevent depression

Help you concentrate better

Help in creativity

Help you to live longer

Improve memory

Reduce inflammation in the body

Help prevent circles under the eyes

You will have better relationships with family members, coworkers and others.

Symptoms of insomnia

Difficulty falling asleep (lying awake in bed for an hour or more tossing and turning wishing to fall asleep).

Waking up during the night and have trouble falling asleep again.

Waking up too early in the morning.

Feeling tired, irritable, exhausted, and anxious during the day.

Not feeling rested after a night's sleep.

Increased accidents or errors

Worrying about not being able to sleep

Depression and or anxiety.

Difficulty focusing on tasks, paying attention.

Forgetfulness

Causes of insomnia

Worrying: This is probably one of the most reasons why people don't sleep. They worry about anything from what they will eat for breakfast to how they will pay their rent/mortgage, health, family, money and everything in between. "How many times have you been worrying about something that never happened?"

Work: Many people carry their work to bed with them; they constantly relive what they should have done and did not do or what they did that should not have been done. After they will start another dialogue of what they will or won't do tomorrow.

Foods: Caffeine as additive foods…chocolate, milk chocolate pudding, chocolate mousse, chocolate frostings, in fact anything with chocolate.

Drinks: with caffeine such as coffee, tea, some herbal teas, cocoa, sodas, alcohol, energy drinks, chocolate, even some over the counter medicines and some ice creams.

Health: Cardiovascular disease, low thyroid function, kidney disease, neurological disorders, pain (acute or chronic), mental health, diabetes, musculoskeletal disorders such as arthritis or fibromyalgia, heartburn, depression, anxiety, stress, restless leg syndrome, sleep apnea, pregnancy .

Stress: job, finances, divorce, relocating, travelling, taking care of other family members.

Environment: the temperature of your bedroom…is it too hot or too cold, is it noisy, do you read/watch TV or eat in bed, if you have a partner, is he/she snoring a problem. Before going to bed do you say to yourself that you are going to have difficulty sleeping or falling asleep, if you do then you are setting yourself up for another sleepless night.

Mattress/pillows: are these comfortable or do they need replacing, is your mattress too hard or too soft. All these things can set you up for not sleeping well.

Eating: just before going to bed may cause you to feel uncomfortable or you may have heartburn which will make it difficult to fall asleep.

Menopause: about 80% of women going through menopause have trouble sleeping due to having hot flashes.

Pain: According to the National Sleep Foundation 21% of American suffer from chronic pain which cause loss of sleep, and 36% have acute pain. When people suffer from pain their sleep is affected. People who suffer from pain also suffer from about getting a good night sleep.

Types of insomnia

There are 3 types of insomnia:

Primary and secondary.

Primary insomnia is when a person is having sleep problems that is not related to a health problem.

Secondary insomnia is having problems sleeping due to either a health condition, medications they are taking or the use of substances such as alcohol or drugs.

There is acute, chronic and transient insomnia.

Acute insomnia: is the inability to sleep well consistently for a period of less than a month due to:

Sickness of any kind

Pain

Stress…divorce

Death of loved one

Loss of job

Moving

Children

Caring for other family members etc.

Medications that treat allergies, colds, ADHD, asthma may interfere with sleep.

Environmental situations such as being extremely hot or cold, noise, light which may cause you to not sleep.

Physical or emotional discomfort.

Shift changes.

Travel

Bad news

Allergies/sinuses

Often time's acute insomnia can resolve on its own without any treatment.

Chronic insomnia is having problems sleeping due to either a health condition, medications they are taking or the use of substances such as alcohol or drugs lasts longer than a month can include:

Chronic physical pain.

Stress over a period of time

Uncomfortable mattress/pillow

Depression/anxiety

Transient insomnia: lasts for less than a week, can be caused by another disorder, or by sleep environment.
Injury
Surgery
Travelling
Loss of a loved one
Acute illness
Loss of a job
Exams

Stages of sleep: when we sleep there is still a lot going on inside your head that is responsible for the different stages of sleep.

There are 2 main types of sleep

1. Non-Rapid eye movement (known as quiet sleep)

2. Rapid eye movement (known as active sleep)

There are 4 stages of sleep…

Stage 1 is the first stage when you are in a light stage of sleep. A transition between wakefulness and sleep. This period last for about 5 to 10 minutes. If you wake someone while they are in this stage they may tell you they really were not asleep.

Stage 2 lasts for about 20 minutes. The brain starts to produce bursts of rapid, rhythmic brain wave activity and the body temperature starts to decrease.

Stage 3 in this stage there is deep slow brain waves known as delta waves. During this stage you are less responsive and not hear activities and noises going on around you.

Stage 4 this is known as the rapid eye movement sleep. This stage is characterized by increased respiration rate, eye movement and increased brain activity. Muscles become more relaxed and dreaming occurs due to brain activity.

When to see a doctor?

If you have a health problem that is causing your insomnia you should visit your doctor, sometimes there may a health problem that you are not aware of and your doctor can run some tests or have you do a sleep study. Whether or not you have a medical problem, if you are having many sleepless nights you should still see your doctor who may be able to help you understand why you are having difficulty sleeping.

How is insomnia diagnosed?

If you think you have insomnia you should talk to your doctor. He/she may need to perform an evaluation which may include a physical examination including a medical history to rule out any health issues you may be having.

The doctor may ask questions such as:

A history of your sleep patterns

How long does it take you to fall asleep?

How often do you wake up during the night and how long it takes for you to fall asleep again?

How long have you had this problem and how often?

If you feel tired in the morning or not.

Do feel you have to sleep during the day because you are too tired.

Is there anything that is causing you to worry?

Do you worry about falling asleep or staying asleep?

What medications you might be taking?
Do you eat just before going to bed? Sleep
study may be suggested

What is a sleep study?

A sleep study test records what happens to your body during sleep and what is causing your sleeplessness. Your stages of sleep can also be determined by this study. It monitors your brain waves, heart rate, leg movements and breathing during the night. This is done in a sleep study facility overnight.

Why do a sleep study?

This may be done to find sleep problems such as:

Excessive snoring.

If you have a problem call sleep apnea (when a person stops breathing while asleep for 10 seconds or more.

Narcolepsy (problems staying awake)

Sleepwalking.

Shift work sleep disorder (needing to sleep during the day due to rotating shift work).

Movement of the limbs that you may be unaware of such as the muscles of the arms or feet twitching during sleep.

Preparing for a sleep study test?

On the day of your appointment you should make sure and wash your hair including having a shower, do not put anything on your hair or creams/lotions on your body, avoid any caffeine drinks after breakfast, you may want to take some reading material with you or a video to watch, you should also have something to eat before leaving for your appointment. When you arrive you will be met by a technologist at about 7pm who will show you to your room to get changed preferably in a 2 piece pajamas after taking your information. You need to take your own pajamas.

The technician will then hook you up to some electrodes and sensors which will remain overnight and they will monitor the activities. Yes! I know because I've been through it. Take any medications that you are now taking with you. You should also keep a record of your sleep habit for a few days before going for your appointment and take it with you.

Patients are woken up between 5:30 and

6am for the equipment to be removed. This takes approximately 15 minutes. If you need to wake up earlier let the technician know.

The result will be sent to your doctor and you will be notified.

Sleep disorders

Acute and chronic pain

Restless leg syndrome

Sleep apnea

Certain medications

Teeth grinding

Fibromyalgia

Allergies

Asthma

Difficulty breathing

Heart disease

GERD (heartburn)

Pregnancy

ADHD

Narcolepsy – excessive daytime sleepiness

Being sick

Mental illness

Post traumatic stress disorder

Panic attacks

Depression

Difficulty focusing

Dangers of too little sleep

More and more people are sacrificing hours of sleep to either fit in more activities, more working hours or more hours of TV and video games without realizing the dangers of having insufficient sleep can cause to your health.

Dangers of too little sleep are:

Increased risk of getting into a motor vehicle accident

Accidents while working on machinery

You are at risk for being overweight

Diabetes

Depression

Heart attacks

Strokes

Thinking ability

Memory

Forgetful

Learning

Judgment

Loss of interest in sex

Irritability

Anxiety

Tiredness

Headache

Immune system

Blood pressure

Moody

Low energy

Tripping over things

Can also affect your relationship with family members and coworkers.

Cheating yourself of sleep can also lead to damage of the heart, brain and kidneys over a period of time.

Over-the-counter sleep medications:

Many people who are having problems to sleep go to the pharmacy and buy over-the-counter medicines to help them sleep but there are other things you should know about this.

Benadryl and Unisom: are sedating antihistamines. The side effects may include drowsiness during the day, dry mouth, constipation, blurred vision etc.

Melatonin: helps to control your sleep-wake cycle. Side effects can include daytime sleepiness and headache.

Pain medicines: some pain medicines may actually help you to sleep such as PM Tylenol, Advil and Motrin.

Over-the-counter medications should be taken for short periods. You need to talk to the pharmacist or your doctor if you are taking any prescription medicines as some of them may counteract each other.

Sleeping pills do not cure the underlying cause of your sleep problems, but can even make the problem worse.

Side effects of over the counter medications;

Drowsy the next day,

Tired

Blurred vision

Dry mouth

Forgetfulness

Feeling off balance

Before using any sleep aids for children under 12 years, women who are pregnant or the elderly you should seek medical advice from your doctor first.

Prescription medicines: there are many medications that are prescribed by your doctor to help you sleep. Before the doctor gives you a prescription for something to help you sleep you should let the doctor know all the medications and any herbal supplements you are using and also what the side effects would be for the medication he/she is prescribing. **Some prescription medications for sleep are**:

These are some of the more commonly used ones:

Ambien: this is a sedative and may impair your thinking or reactions. You may also still feel sleepy in the morning.

Lunesta: help you to fall asleep quickly and get seven to eight hours of sleep. If you cannot get this amount of sleep you should not take it since it may cause you to feel groggy in the morning.

Halcion, Zanax, Restoril may stay in your system longer but may cause you to feel sleepy during the day. You can also become dependent on these drugs because you may always need them to help you sleep.

Supplements:

Valerian" reduces the amount of time it takes you to fall asleep but it takes a few weeks to see results.

Melatonin: this supplement regulates the normal sleep/wake cycle. Many people use this supplement.

Nightrest: this is a formula that has a soothing effect on the body and mind and helps the body to relax and go off to sleep. **It worked the very first night I took it.**

Magnesium and calcium: this supplement helps to maintain normal muscle and nerve function. Several older studies show that magnesium can improve the quality of your sleep.

5HTP: this is an amino-acid and is created naturally in the body which helps to make serotonin. This is a chemical in the brain and controls your mood.

Theanine: is an amino acid found in green tea calms the neurotransmitters in the brain reduce anxiety and promote relaxation.

Simple changes:

Worry: Be logical and realize that worry cannot help the condition about which you are worrying. With a troubled mind and very little sleep will rob you of the stamina which could help you to combat the causes of your worry.

Write down your worries on a paper or notebook and steps you can take to solve them.

A philosopher once wrote "Most worry is a lie," "Seldom do the things you worry about materialize," he added. Think of the many things you have worried about in the past and you will agree with this wise man.

When you prepare to go bed instead of worrying think "while I am asleep my subconscious mind will find a solution to my problem."

Before retiring at night, take a few moments and review the day's work. If there is anything that did not please you, decide what you will do about it the following day or in the future. Know that a good night's rest will let you awaken in the morning refreshed and ready to start a great day of accomplishment.

Electronic gadgets: turn off your electronic gadgets including sending emails. Your brain gets revved up instead of calming down. The glow from the electronic gadgets works against quality sleep. Have a transition period of about thirty minutes before going to bed.

Use your bed for only 2 things:

1. Sleep

2. Making love

That's it.

Deep breathing: sometimes just breathing deeply for a few minutes can release tension and clear your mind. When you feel tense and anxious you tend to breathe shallow which limits your oxygen intake.

Sit up straight or lie down. Exhale completely through your mouth. Place your hand on your stomach or place a book on your stomach, breath in slowly through your nose and let your stomach rise (notice your hand or the book will push outwards Hold your breath to a count of five if you can handle it, then slowly contract your stomach till most of the air is out. Try this for a few minutes.

Foods: Foods to help you fall asleep: a chemical found in certain foods called tryptophan help you to sleep, when broken down in the body it produces serotonin. Foods with serotonin are turkey, fish, red meat, poultry, shrimp, and eggs, milk, bananas, mangoes, nuts and seeds especially pumpkin seeds, sunflower seeds, walnuts, almonds, lentils kidney and black beans.

Drinks: Refrain from caffeine drinks late in the day or foods with caffeine including alcohol, although some people can fall asleep after having cup of coffee. A cup of warm milk with a teaspoon of honey added helps you to relax and fall asleep.

Bedroom: mattress/pillows: you need to be sure your mattress and pillows are comfortable. After all we spend one third of our lives in bed. Do not read; eat watch TV or play electronic or board games in bed. Turn of your electronic gadgets at least an hour before you are ready to retire and start dimming the lights. All these things can set you up for not sleeping well. Make sure you are not too warm or too cold or that your bed is situated in an area where there is a draft.

Milk: I am sure everyone has heard about drinking a cup of warm milk before retiring helps you to sleep. The fact is this does not work for everyone. So try adding a teaspoon of honey in a glass of warm milk some people say it help them drift off to sleep due to its calming effect.

Music: calming music help to induce sleep at night. Music is safe and does not have any side effects. Some people like listening to calming music, others to nature music and still others like listening to music such as Mozart and Tchaikovsky.

Sleep pillow: this is very simple to make. With a piece of cloth 4 inches by 8 inches or you can use a larger piece of cloth. Mix ¼ cup lavender flowers, ¼ cup mugwort and ¼ cup hops blend these together. Fold the cloth in half and sew 2 sides leaving 1 side to fill the sack. Fill the mixture in the sack and sew up the other end. Place inside your pillow case when you go to bed. You will have a restful night sleep.

Special box: You can also have a special box where you can wrap your worries when you retire and safely place it in this box till the next day when you wake up, or place your worries in a balloon and let it fly away.

Relaxing: create time to relax before going to bed. You can just squeeze a soft ball and relax your hands for a few minutes or sip a cup of tea. Use the thumb and forefinger to massage the soft area between the thumb and index finger.

Exercises and sleep: exercise significantly improves the sleep of people with chronic insomnia. A number of sleep studies have discovered that daytime exercise promotes better sleep. Even walking 1 mile as an older adult can help your sleep cycle. There are many different types of exercises such as dancing aerobics, cycling, swimming etc. The important thing is to start and continue doing it.

Noises: If after 20 minutes or so of lying in bed and not being able to sleep you should get up and read a book or listen to some soft music. If noise is an issue you may want to use earplugs or use a fan which will help drown out some of the noise. If there are any unavoidable sounds or noises which may keep you awake, get the right attitude toward the sounds instead of resenting them and they'll no longer bother you. Perhaps you live in a neighborhood where there is considerable street noise. Resenting it will keep you awake. Learn to be indifferent toward the many sounds, and you will soon forget them.

Hot shower or bath: with some aromatherapy oils can help relax the body and help you fall asleep. Roman chamomile or Lavender is a good one.
Acupressure: this is an ancient technique where you use your fingers to press certain points on your body which stimulates natural healing. In the first indentation below the outer ankle, and just below the inside of the

ankle bone there is a slight indentation. Massage both these points together for a few minutes. Massage legs, one then the other.

Hold your hand in front of you with palm facing upwards locate this pressure point in the crease of your wrist in line with your little finger and massage for a few minutes using moderate pressure and slow circular movements.

Beneath the ball of your foot is a pressure point that can help you relax and get to sleep more easily. Use your thumb to apply pressure, and gently massage this area until you feel very calm and restful.

There are several techniques to do this and no one is wrong, chose the one that you feel comfortable doing. There are also many CD's on the market for sale on meditation and visualization; you can also borrow them from libraries. You will find that as you continue to do this you will eventually start feeling better.

Meditation: How to meditate? If you are someone who does meditation on a regular basis, please continue; if you have

never tried meditation before don't think you have to sit in a certain position for any length of time. Meditation is a technique that has been practiced.

In the East for thousands of years and there are several different ways to do it. It restores your internal balance and stimulates the immune system.

Take at least 5 minutes twice a day or longer periods if you have the time and sit in a quiet area undisturbed area. The important thing is you try to do it regular.

Sit upright without leaning against the wall a chair back or anything, you don't have to sit with your legs crossed. You can also sit on a chair. Sit comfortably with your back straight so it will be helpful when breathing,

Sit upright on a chair with both feet touching the floor.

Close your eyes or open them a little.

Relax your arms and legs; you can also rest your hands on your lap, the important thing is to keep your spine straight.

Follow your breath in and out and count it as one breath, count to 10 and start from one again.

Breathing in and out counts as one breathe, or you can recite a Mantra which is a word such as OHM, LOVE, PEACE or whatever else you would like to use as a mantra or visualize something or some place that calms you. You will find there are many thoughts that come up, don't push the thoughts away, just acknowledge them and let them go by.

Many thoughts will come up but you just need There are several techniques to do this and no one is wrong, chose the one that you feel comfortable doing. There are also many CD's on the market for sale on meditation and visualization; you can also borrow them from libraries. You will find that as you continue to do this you will eventually start feeling better.

Guided imagery: are pictures that one imagines. You can practice this alone, with the help of someone who knows how to do guided imagery or with a CD which can be

bought at stores like some Wal-Mart, Target, Barnes and Noble or online

Pain: if you have health problems including

chronic pain you should seek the help of your doctor even though you may not think you have a health problem the doctor will be able to do some simple test to determine if your thyroid or adrenals play a part in your sleeplessness.

If after 20 minutes or so of lying in bed and not being able to sleep you should get up and read a book or listen to some soft music or do some meditation.

Teas

Teas: many people like having a cup of tea before going to bed it helps them to unwind from their daily activities and help them to relax. Does tea really help you to sleep? There is not much evidence that teas have a sedative effect yet millions of people swear that it works.

So here is a list of teas:
Chamomile: is the tea that most people

drink to help them sleep. You can make it yourself by drying out the flowers and then brewing it or you can purchase the ones that are sold in grocery stores and health food shops. Other uses are it can be applied to the skin and mucus membrane for inflammation, parasitic worms, and sore throats and to sooth anal or genital inflammation.

Side effects: Do NOT use if you are allergic to ragweed pollens. Avoid during pregnancy or if using any blood thinners such as Warfarin or Cyclosporine.

Lemon balm: is from the mint family believed to help you relax and so aid in helping you fall asleep. Other uses are it helps with digestive problems, flatulence, vomiting, headache, toothache and pain.

Side effects: no known side effects but should be take for a three week period then come off it for a week then repeat.

Valerian: this herb has actually been found to have a sedative effect. It may take anywhere from 2 to 4 weeks to feel the effect. The tea is made from the root of the flower or you can

purchase them in the supermarkets or health food shops. It enhances the quality of your sleep and you do not feel groggy when you wake up. Other uses of valerian are it eases stomach and menstrual cramps.

Side effects: although considered safe valerian may cause headaches, dizziness and gastrointestinal problems. Avoid this herb if you are pregnant or breast feeding or have liver disease. Do not take if using other drugs for depression or alcohol.

Passionflower: passionflower is usually combined with other herbs and helps you to sleep. Other uses of passionflower are gastrointestinal upset related to nervousness or anxiety, asthma, fibromyalgia, attention deficit-hyperactivity disorder, high blood pressure.

Avoid using this herb if you are pregnant because it stimulates the uterine. Side effects: No side effects have been noted but use in moderation. Do not take passionflower or any other herbs if you are already using prescription medications for

anxiety or depression. This can result in excessive sleepiness.

Hops: has a sedating effect and is used for sleep. It has a bitter aromatic taste and is used to flavor and preserve beer. **Side effects:** no side effects have been noted when used in moderation. **If you are using any type of prescription drugs or using alcohol, if you are pregnant or nursing also Some people have allergies to various herbs so talk to a health professional before using any herbs, aromatherapy or supplements..**

Aromatherapy: is the use of essential oils which is derived from plants known as essential oils and is used for the treatment or prevention of disease. It is a complementary therapy which treats not only the symptoms but the person as a whole.

Essential oils can be used to massage the body, as aromatherapy using a diffuser, in the bath water, can be used as a spray on your pillow or in your room, can also be massaged at the temples, at the bottom of your feet or even dab a little on your night light in your room. The aromas from these oils are very soothing and relaxing some even have a sedative effect.

These oils have to be diluted before applying to the body. Can be diluted with a carrier oil such as olive oil, coconut oil, jojoba oil and almond oil. Many people have sensitivity toward essential oils.

Care must be taken when using any essential oils. If you are pregnant, breast feeding, have allergies, sensitivity or compromised immune deficiency talk you a health practitioner before using.

There are many different types of essential oils that can be used for different situations.

Here are a few essential oils:

Lavender: studies have been shown that lavender aids with sleep it is cheap and nontoxic. You can buy a pillow filled with lavender or you can get a spray bottle and spray some on your pillow or in your room before going to bed. It can also be used for burns, calming yourself or others, bee stings, hand creams and lotions, shampoos, or just to soak your feet.

Ylang Ylang: this essential oil has a sedative effect and can also be used as an antiseptic and antispasmodic.

Marjoram: most people use it for cooking but it also in getting a peaceful night sleep and rubbing into sore joints and muscles.

Roman chamomile: it has a light floral scent and is great for creating a peaceful atmosphere in your bedroom. It has calming, relaxing and soothing properties.

Cedar wood oil: has many health benefits

including a sedative effect. It also has a soothing and calming effect on the mind.

You may need to take medications to help you sleep due to some health problem or to get you through a few nights that is fine. If you have a chronic sleep problem and you do not know what the problem is you should seek the help of your doctor or someone who can determine the underlying cause. Only when you know the underlying cause you will be able to treat your insomnia properly.

Summary

Here is what we learned from this book. We learned the benefits of sleeping well, signs symptoms of insomnia, causes of insomnia, when to see a doctor and how insomnia is diagnosed and treated. Sleep disorders and the dangers of not sleeping well

We also learned about over the counter medicines and prescriptions medicines but most of all we learned how to make simple changes that can have you sleeping well for a long long time.

Changes such as exercising, not eating a heavy meal just before retiring for bed, not using your computer or anything that has a screen light at least one hour before bedtime. Give yourself time to wind down from the day, write down your worries so you would be able to deal with it the next day. Do some relaxing exercises or meditation, listen to soft music or use some aromatherapy, have a hot bath or shower before going to bed. Have a cup of herbal non-caffeine tea or use a sleep-pillow.

Making changes will cost you either nothing

or very little money, but may cost you a little time.

Resources

The American Sleep Apnea Association
1717 Pennsylvania Avenue, NW Ste. 1025
Washington, DC 20006
Ph. 1-888-293-3650

www.sleepapnea.org

National Sleep Foundation
1010 N. Glebe Road, Ste. 310
Arlington, VA 22201
Ph. 703-243-1697

Email: nsf@sleepfoundation.org
www.sleepfoundation.org

American Academy of Sleep Medicine
2510 North Frontage Road
Darien, IL 60561
Ph. 630-737-9700
www.aasmnet.org

Narcolepsy Network, Inc.
129 Waterwheel Lane
North Kingstown, RI 02852
Ph. 401-667-2523
Email: narnet@narcolepsynetwork.org
www.narcolepsynetwork.org

National Sleep Foundation1
1010 N. Glebe Road
Suite 310
Arlington, VA 22201 USA
Phone **703**)243-1697
E-mail nsf@sleepfoundation.org
www.sleepfoundation.com

NHLBI Health Information Center
P.O. Box 30105
Bethesda, MD 20824-0105

nhlbiinfo@nhlbi.nih.gov

301-592-8573

I Can Make You Sleep by Paul McKenna

www.ingramcontent.com/pod-product-compliance
Lightning Source LLC
Chambersburg PA
CBHW070820290526
45795CB00002B/789